Fighting Fatigue

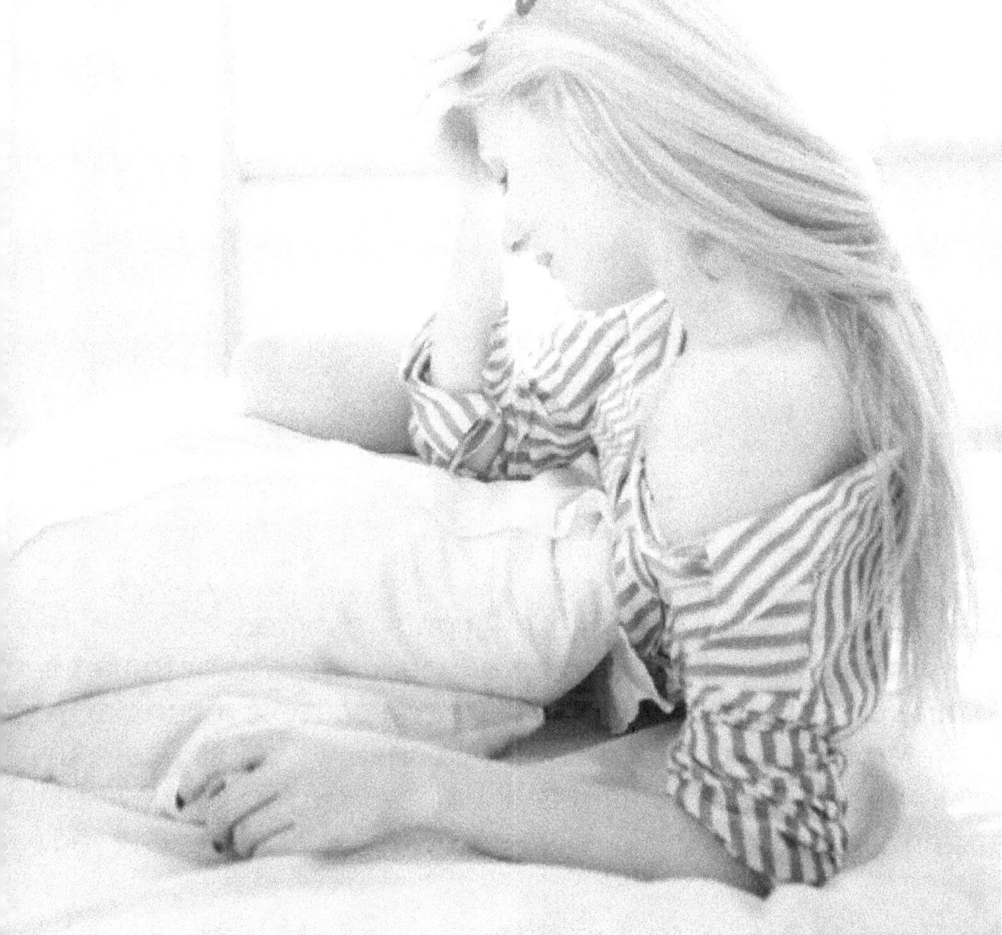

DANI HONEYCUTT

Fighting Fatigue

How to Take Back Your Life by Overcoming Fatigue

By Dani Honeycutt

DISCLAIMER:

This information is not presented by a medical practitioner and is for educational and informational purposes only. The content is not intended to be a substitute for professional medical advice, diagnosis, or treatment. Always seek the advice of your physician or other qualified healthcare provider with any questions you may have regarding a medical condition. Never disregard professional medical advice or delay in seeking it because of something you have read.

Contents

Foreword

I have been fighting fatigue for as long as I can remember. Even as a child, I used to love to take naps and never skipped the opportunity to lay down for as much sleep as I could get. Every Sunday, we would go to church as a family then gather at my maternal grandparents for a massive family dinner. I come from a large family, so there were always fifteen or more people there for dinner. After I ate my grandmother's amazing southern cooking, I needed to sleep some of those calories off. Sunday after Sunday, you could find my grandfather asleep in his recliner and I was asleep on the couch. I have always been a nap person. Any day, any time.

In my early twenties, I was diagnosed with hypothyroidism which explained several things. But my health didn't stop declining regardless of being on medication for hypothyroidism. MayoClinic.org explains, "Hypothyroidism (underactive thyroid) is a condition in which your thyroid gland doesn't produce enough of certain crucial hormones. Hypothyroidism may not cause noticeable symptoms in the early stages. Over time, untreated hypothyroidism can cause a number of health problems, such as obesity, joint pain, infertility and heart disease."

In my late twenties, I was diagnosed with PCOS, which is polycystic ovary syndrome. It comes with its own set of symptoms and worries. In my early thirties, I started being diagnosed with autoimmune diseases, one of which is

Hashimoto's. In layman's terms, my immune system is attacking and killing my thyroid.

The thyroid gland controls more than you may think. From hormones to regulating body temperature, thyroid function can determine how I feel from one day to the next. The thyroid gland is part of your endocrine system, which produces hormones that coordinate many of your body's functions.

MayoClinic.org lists signs and symptoms of hypothyroidism include:

- Fatigue and sluggishness
- Increased sensitivity to cold
- Constipation
- Pale, dry skin
- A puffy face
- Brittle nails
- Hair loss
- Enlargement of the tongue
- Unexplained weight gain
- Muscle aches, tenderness and stiffness
- Joint pain and stiffness
- Muscle weakness
- Excessive or prolonged menstrual bleeding
- Depression
- Memory lapses

I am currently undergoing tests to see if I have progressed to a lupus diagnosis.

All of these are health related reasons for a lifetime of fatigue. Sometimes, the battle feels overwhelming. I encourage you not to let it bring you down. It can get better for you. As many things in life, the fatigue will ebb and flow. Just as surely as the dawn follows the night, your fatigue will lift. Do not stop living life. You can safely so "no" to some things without forfeiting your dreams and goals.

You are enough. You are amazing. You are more than how you feel. You can find a way to overcome your challenges, just as I have. You are a superhero.

Many people are walking around, driving, going to work and living their lives in a permanent state of fatigue. Sometimes people are tired for unexplained health reasons, but often there are typical reasons for fatigue which include lack of regular sleep, poor diet, and not getting enough exercise. Fatigue can be very frustrating and even disabling due to feeling as if you cannot get things done or enjoy your downtime.

In this book, we're going to look at different ways to combat and overcome fatigue so that you can get your life back. There is no reason to be tired all the time. It's not a normal state of being in healthy people. If you use all these ideas there is no doubt that you're going to be on your way to not just getting over fatigue, but also becoming an energetic, happy, recharged individual who can accomplish more than you ever thought you could.

Why You Feel Exhausted Even on Your Best Days

Before we get into the meat of getting recharged, let's address the fact that sometimes medical issues will play an important role in your energy levels. These can drag you down no matter how well you do on any given day.

If you are suffering from unexplained exhaustion, it's important that you seek medical answers first. Go to your doctor and ask them to give you a complete blood work-up to check all your vitamin and hormone levels, plus test you for common diseases that cause exhaustion like sleep apnea. Alternatively, you may be taking medication for an illness and one of the side effects is tiredness. If you feel tired after taking the medication for two weeks, ask your doctor if there are alternatives.

The following conditions can easily be tested for and acknowledged by your primary care doctor through typical blood tests.

Anemia

This medical condition is characterized by paleness, fatigue, racing heart, and sometimes even upper left quadrant abdominal pain. If a person has anemia their red blood cell count (known as hemoglobin) is too low. If hemoglobin gets too low, it can cause severe fatigue and other problems as well. For men, hemoglobin levels less than 13.5 grams per 100 ml and for women, hemoglobin less than 12.0 grams per 100 ml is too low.

Other Vitamin Deficiencies

Besides low iron, if you are short on vitamins D3 or B12 you may feel severely fatigued and even anxious, which can cause you to lose sleep - thus making you feel even more tired all day long. Even though you can buy D3 and B12 (with folate) to help with this issue, it is still best to get a blood test to rule out anything serious before starting with treatment.

Thyroid Disease

Whether you're hypothyroid (slow) or hyperthyroid (fast), you will suffer from fatigue. Having said that, hypothyroidism tends to cause you to feel tired, sluggish, and even depressed, while hyperthyroidism tends to make people feel anxious, restless, irritable and then contribute to fatigue due to lack of sleep. If you are feeling tired even if you have bursts of energy, ask your doctor to test your thyroid levels to be on the safe side.

Diabetes

One of the biggest first indications of diabetes is fatigue. Even though most people think diabetes only affects overweight people, many people who appear healthy still wind up with type II diabetes.

If you already know you have diabetes and are often tired, talk to your doctor about this. Today, even older people are being diagnosed with type I diabetes, so the old rules don't fit anymore. You can feel fatigued whether your blood sugar is high or low; if it's off you will feel the effects. That's why it's so important to talk to your doctor to try to manage your disease through medication, diet, exercise, and regular sleep.

Depression and Anxiety

While there can be underlying causes of depression and anxiety such as anemia and other vitamin and mineral deficiencies, sometimes people have these conditions for other or even unknown reasons. If you've checked everything and nothing shows up, talk to a professional about whether you suffer from depression or anxiety (or both). Anxiety causes fatigue by preventing a good night's rest, and depression sometimes has the effect of making you want to sleep away your problems regardless of how much sleep you get.

Chronic Fatigue Syndrome

Another illness that can cause fatigue is CFS. It's right in the name. There could be many causes for CFS that we don't know yet. But it is a real medical condition that is often characterized by fever, body aches, and protracted exhaustion. This condition sometimes occurs after you think you're recovered from another viral infection. It's very difficult to diagnose and is only given after a complete work-up to discount other possibilities. But it is a real illness that can be managed and treated.

Sleep Apnea

An almost epidemic problem today, sleep apnea is caused by either an obstruction due to the way you sleep, or because the brain isn't signaling your muscles to breathe properly even if your airway isn't blocked (known as central sleep apnea). Both types of apnea are very dangerous and can lead to sudden death while sleeping. However, most often what it leads to is a low quality of life due to experiencing non-restorative sleep.

To diagnose this issue, you'll be sent to a sleep center overnight to do a sleep study. There are many ways to get help with this problem. Even if no one has mentioned that you snore, this is a great test to get to ensure that you are sleeping well.

Medications

If you have any type of illness where you've been given medications, they may be causing your problems. They might make you tired, or they may make it hard for you to sleep - thus causing daytime fatigue. Sometimes you still must take the medication, but often there are other options that you can use so that you can find a medication that doesn't cause you as many problems. Other times, there are additional medications that you can take to combat the problem if it's interfering with your ability to live your life fully.

So, now that we have talked about potential medical issues that cause fatigue, we can move on to talk about other issues that may cause fatigue and how you can overcome it. After all, the entire point is to find ways to recharge your body and take control of your life. Whether that is via medical intervention or something else is less important than doing something to make a difference.

How Mental Exhaustion Affects the Whole Body

Everyone thinks it's normal for someone to be tired if they work out in a field all day or stand on their feet all day. People who have a desk job or spend a lot of their time on mental tasks are often surprised and shocked that they are still exhausted.

Mental exhaustion can affect your entire body in negative ways. Not only are people with mental exhaustion tired, they also often suffer from body aches as if they have worked out all day long. Overusing your mind is just as bad for you as overusing yourself physically.

For example, many people who suffer from mental exhaustion, in addition to being tired most of the time, may start to get sick more often, have a lot of headaches, experience back pain, muscle aches and more. Plus, mental exhaustion can affect your ability to get a good night's sleep which can just make all the above worse.

Take note of the symptoms that are caused by mental exhaustion. If you have more than a few of these and have been burning the wick at both ends, consider mental exhaustion a potential culprit.

- Constant sleepiness
- Frequent headaches
- Hallucinations
- Impaired decision making
- Inability to concentrate and focus
- Irritability
- Loss of appetite
- Memory problems
- Moodiness
- Muscle weakness
- Poor coordination
- Poor judgement
- Reduced immunity
- Slow reflexes
- Sore or aching muscles
- Unexplained dizziness
- Unmotivated

When people are mentally exhausted, their body tries to get them to take a break and rest in every way it can. That's why it's so important to pay attention to the signs of mental exhaustion. Thankfully, there are ways to combat and overcome mental exhaustion, which we will discuss next.

How to Overcome Mental Exhaustion

Suffering from mental exhaustion is not a fun experience. It can sneak up on you. You may think you're doing wonderfully well and then one day you realize you're not. Let's go through some steps to overcome mental exhaustion but also learn how to prevent it in the first place. After all, prevention is the best medicine.

- Track How You Spend Your Time – If you don't know how much you're really doing, it can be easy to just keep going 24/7 and never take a break. Take some time to track what you're doing daily for about a week. You can use your smartphone to track your activities or you can go old school and carry around a small notebook to record your activities in.

- Drop Activities That Don't Produce Real Results – When you look at the activities you did while tracking, note the things that aren't really producing results, or that are busy work, or that are completely unnecessary. For example, do you go to a lot of meetings? Do you have to? Do you spend a lot of time trying to help a relative, friend, or someone else without results? Let go of anything that you can either just stop doing or outsource. Or if you must keep doing it, find a way to put limits on it.

- Put Everything in Your Calendar – One reason people get overscheduled doing too much and become mentally exhausted is that they think they're magic. They think they can do 48 hours of work in 24 hours. But, if you started putting everything on your calendar properly, you would see that you just can't. First, schedule the must-dos. Then add in family time, date night, friend time, and "me" time to your day. Don't add anything to your schedule that will reduce these important things.

- Get a Good Night's Sleep – Don't forget how important sleep is. Most adults should seek to get between six and nine hours a night. It largely depends on your genetics how much sleep feels right for you. Work with what you know you need. If you're having trouble sleeping at night, address that issue so that you fall asleep fast and your sleeping time is productive. To help get used to this process, go to bed and wake up at the same time every day for at least 30 days. You can start with the least time and work your way up to find out which amount of time works best for you to make you feel rested each day.

- Exercise Every Day – Schedule in exercise time each day. It doesn't have to be strenuous exercise. It can be as simple as a brisk walk. You also don't need to schedule in an entire hour. Look at your schedule so that you can determine if you have 10 minutes to walk six times a day, or three 20-minute walks a day. You can also separate that out into different types of exercise. The important thing is to get up out of a chair and move as much as you can. I personally love to play video games. So, I purchased "Just Dance" and I play it on the console that I have. I enjoy getting to play the game and it even has a "sweat mode" for more of a cardio workout.

- Eat Right – Enough cannot be stated about eating the right type of food for your body. What you eat often depends on what you need. Ask your doctor to test your blood levels for vitamins and then eat the things you need to avoid deficiencies. Try eating smaller meals throughout the day which will give you a break, boost your energy, and help you stay more focused.

- Stay Hydrated – It can be very easy to get dehydrated. Most adults should drink between eight and ten 8-ounce glasses of water each day to stay hydrated. If you exercise strenuously, you'll need more. Tea, coffee, soda, and sugary drinks (even fake sugar) are all dehydrating and don't do the same thing as clean, filtered water will. Take the challenge and commit to drinking enough water for 30 days, and you'll see a huge difference.

- Take Regular Breaks – When you are doing mental tasks, it's hard to want to take a break sometimes because there are times when the time is just flying by as you work, and you just don't notice. It is imperative that you take regular breaks. Since the brain works in 90-minute cycles, one way to accomplish breaks is to set up five- to ten-minute breaks every 115 minutes. Set a timer if you must. Get up and stretch, go for a fast walk, grab a snack, drink some water, and you'll come back refreshed.

- Rest Your Eyes – Many people who are using their brains all day tend to sit in front of a computer. Computer monitors are very bad for your eyes. You can install software such as f.lux (https://justgetflux.com) to help lessen the strain but getting away from the monitor on your regular breaks is going to help too.

- Understand That It's OK to Do Nothing – A lot of smart, busy people tend to be uncomfortable with downtime. They feel as if they're slackers. Even if you have a mentally exhausting job as compared to a physically exhausting one, everyone needs to get away sometime. Schedule your yearly vacations and do something. Even if you just stay home and look at local sites, that's okay - everyone needs downtime, and everyone needs time to do nothing.

If you are currently mentally exhausted due to a project of some kind, and if it's possible, take a sick day on a Friday or Monday, or take two vacation days - one on a Friday and one on a Monday. Spend that time resting, doing nothing,

eating right, drinking water, and just getting yourself back.
Then start fresh when you go back to work or school.

Activities That Raise Your Physical and Mental Energy Levels

There are many activities that you can do to help raise your energy level, whether you need more mental energy or physical energy. Your mental and physical energy are so intertwined that when you do something to help one, you're automatically helping the other. Here are some effective activities to try.

- Develop a Daily Meditation/Prayer Practice – Meditation is an important way to help reduce mental stress so that you can focus better. Not only that; you'll also learn to be more mindful of everything you do, which will help you avoid exhaustion in the first place. If you are a spiritual/religious person, spend this time in prayer if that is what you wish. This often strengthens our relationship with our higher power and allows us to clear our minds for the day.

- Move Your Body Every Single Day – Moving is something that is so important that even if you have a physical job, you should still find a way to get in more moving in an intentional way. Even if it's just a few brisk ten-minute walks, it's a way to clear your mind and get your blood flowing. Anytime you feel a slump coming on, take a fast walk.

- Keep a Gratitude Journal – Another way to stay energetic, both mentally and physically, is to be a positive person. Not everyone is positive naturally, but you can start to trick your mind into being that way by keeping a gratitude journal. Each night before bed, write down three things you're grateful for. That will make it the last thing you think of each night. You can make this even more effective if you use a journal that is also a coloring book. Coloring will soothe your mind and relax you.

- Find Your Energy Music – Everyone has positive, uplifting music that they really enjoy and that makes them feel upbeat. However, some of it can also make you unproductive, so it's important to try out different types of music for different activities. If you think a song you sing might not be the right one for work, it may very well be just the ticket for your ride home in the car.

- Play a Game – Games and puzzles are great ways to have some downtime but are also good for your mind. Do at least one type of puzzle each day (such as a crossword puzzle) to help keep your brain thinking and to get your mind off other things that are pressuring you and sucking your energy. Sometimes it's fun to play a game with another person too, such as a silly fast card game like Uno just to break the pace.

- Start a Yoga Practice – One of the best exercises for both mind and body is yoga. There are all types of yoga that you can get involved in. If you're a member of Amazon Prime, you can get free videos for beginners to get started. Alternatively, you can join a class, which is a great way to feel more connected to the world at the same time.

- Drink Water and Eat Chocolate – Sometimes, it's impossible to take time out to do anything mentioned. If that's the case, a fast way to improve your energy is to drink water so that you're hydrated and eat a small serving of real, low-sugar chocolate. If you cannot eat chocolate, another alternative is a crunchy apple.

It might seem like these activities will take away from the time you need to spend on things you need to do. But the truth is, the more productive you are, the easier everything will be. Productivity doesn't mean that you need to take more time doing something. It means that you need to focus closely on what's at hand, and not what's to come. By taking breaks with these activities, you can help yourself become far more productive and reduce mental and physical exhaustion exponentially.

Revitalizing Foods to Boost Your Energy All Day

One of the best ways to treat any type of exhaustion, beside hydration, is by eating the right type of food so that you can keep your energy balanced all day long. One thing to understand about food is that it's all just different nutrients.

When you think of food as nutrients, you realize very fast that some things we put into our mouths aren't really food. It's more like a toy, a distraction, or a leisure activity – an unhealthy one at that. For example, coffee and donuts are not nutrients. Therefore, they are a horrible choice for anyone who is suffering from or trying to prevent mental and physical exhaustion.

Understanding that, let's look at some revitalizing foods that you can easily incorporate into your life to help you boost your energy all day. Remember that if you are on a special diet, you can just substitute the ideas so that they fit your way of eating. The important factor is to consider nutrients that give energy.

- Brown Rice – If you normally eat white rice, switch out all your rice to brown rice, or even different colors of wild rice. Rice that has a color and is not processed will be richer in manganese, which is a mineral that helps your body process energy from both carbs and fats better. A good way to cook brown rice is to boil it in salted water just like you do noodles for 20 minutes, drain, then set aside with a lid on for at least 10 more minutes until ready to serve.

- Sweet Potatoes – This is an excellent lunch idea because sweet potatoes are packed with vitamins and minerals. Loaded with vitamin A and C, if you eat a sweet potato for lunch, you'll be much less likely to suffer from the midday slump. They are super-easy to cook in the microwave or bake ahead. You can eat them hot or cold too.

- Bananas – A banana is almost the perfect food. It has plenty of sugar and fiber to slow the digestion of the sugar. You can eat them alone, or you can spread with seed butter like hemp or sunflower seeds to add a protein kick to make it last even longer.

- Apples – This is another naturally fast food. If you buy organic apples you can just wash them off and start eating them as they are. Due to the high fiber in apples, the sugar processes slowly - making them a perfect snack to help you study harder or get over the midday slump at work. If you normally start falling asleep around 3 pm, try grabbing a small apple around 2:30 and you may find that you don't get tired at all.

- Oranges – You know that an orange is high in vitamin C, and of course the hit of sugar will help perk you up too. But the smell of the citrus as you take the time to peel the fruit will also wake you up and give you both a mental and physical boost of energy that can't be beaten. Always eat your oranges rather than juice them for best results.

- Spinach – Everyone knows that spinach is a superfood, but due to its high iron content that is easily digestible by the human body, adding just one cup of spinach to other dishes or smoothies that you eat throughout the day can make a huge difference in your energy levels. Popeye had the right idea, after all. Tip: Adding citrus and a small amount of fruit-based fat like coconut oil or olive oil to your spinach can help your body process the vitamins.

- Eggs – For some people who need more iron and B vitamins but don't want to eat anything that is sugary even if it's a fruit, a boiled egg is the answer. The worries about too much cholesterol isn't a problem for most people and falling asleep or getting overwhelmed due to studying or work can be avoided by adding a boiled egg to your snack options.

- Water – While water isn't a food, it needs to be mentioned. If you're not drinking eight to ten 8-ounce glasses of water each day, look to that as your first reason for exhaustion. Most people are walking around dehydrated and don't even know it. Remember that water is life and the first choice for beverages should always be water.

Adding these foods to your day can make all the difference in the world to your energy levels. When you feel better, you will automatically feel more energetic. In addition to adding these foods to your daily diet, try to eliminate all processed food. Some people also see good results from eliminating dairy from their diets as it can be a cause of congestion, skin issues, and stomach issues for many adults.

How to Rest If You're an Insomniac

For many people, the main reason they are mentally and/or physically exhausted can all come down to issues with sleep. If you are an insomniac, there are steps that you can take to get rest and hopefully reverse your situation.

Seek Medical Assistance

The very first thing anyone with insomnia should do is make a doctor's appointment to talk about the issues. It might help to track the situation using a device like a Fitbit so that you can show your doctor your records. But you can also just write things down, so you don't forget what to talk about with your doctor.

Your doctor should take you seriously and not just automatically prescribe drugs to help you sleep. Even though that might be a short-term answer, it is not a long-term solution. Your doctor will do a complete blood work-up to ensure that you are doing well nutritionally. If you have low iron, B12, or D, these can cause anxiety and insomnia in some people.

Turn Your Bedroom into a Fortress

This is a great excuse to redo your bedroom. Your bedroom should be a sanctuary made for sleeping. Your bed should be the most comfortable that you can afford to buy, along with the sheets and blankets that you use on it.

You may need to test out a few mattresses, but you usually want something that is firmer than you might have thought but also giving. Many types of memory foam mattresses are great for this, as are some of the sleep number type beds.

You can buy good sheets less expensively than you might think if you know what type of sheets you like. Check on Overstock.com and Amazon to find good prices on well-made sheets. The higher thread count, 100 percent cotton sheets are typically the best for most people, as they stay cool and are easy to care for. For blankets, choose layers of blankets instead of one heavy comforter. That way you can adjust as needed for the time of year.

Invest in blackout shades for your windows. You can get them made for your windows at places like Home Depot or Lowe's. They are well worth it. Even if you have a rule with your HOA that they should be white on the back, you can still get blackout shades that will enable you to sleep better at night.

Get a white noise maker too. You can also use a fan if you prefer. The inexpensive box fans make the right type of white noise. It's better to use a white noise that is like a fan or static over sounds of animals or water dripping.

Keep your thermostat set properly. In the winter it should be set on 68 degrees F and in the summer 72. Having a fan to circulate the air is also helpful. If it's nice outside, try opening your window about an hour before you go to bed, but close it if you can when you go to bed so outside noises don't interfere (unless you're lucky enough to live where it's super-quiet or you have the sound of the ocean to lull you to sleep).

Additionally, invest in very comfortable sleeping attire or sleep naked to avoid anything getting in the way of your comfort. If you or your partner snore, consider using comfortable earplugs to help further block the sound. (Suggestion: parents of young children could take turns so every other night at least one parent gets a full night of sleep.)

Turn Off the Lights and Electronics

The darker you can make your room, the better. Once the sun goes down outside, it's important to make the house dimmer too. You want to turn off all electronics at least an hour or two before you go to bed, so that your body gets used to the idea that it's bedtime. That includes your TV, your computer, and your mobile device. This is probably the hardest one for insomniacs to deal with, but it's very important for your health to disconnect.

If you're nervous that something is going to happen to anyone if you're not there immediately, understand that long before there were cell phones, there were parents. Of course, you're going to want to be available to your kids if they're teenagers, but that's what curfews are for and that's why people have two parents. Ask for help and take turns. If you do not have children living at home, you really don't need to be available 24/7 to anyone, most of the time. Anyone who has something to say to you, even if something bad happens, can be dealt with in the morning.

Try it for at least 30 days. You'll see after that time that you're not in charge of the world, and no one needs to bother you about anything when you're sleeping. If you have elderly parents, share the job with your siblings with each of you having assigned "on call" times or something similar so everyone can get sleep. Remember, you cannot take care of others if you don't take care of yourself first.

Start a Bedtime Ritual

A great way to ensure that you get more sleep is to create a bedtime ritual. Since you already need to turn electronics off and turn down the lights, think of something you can do that doesn't require either. For example, soft slow stretches, meditation, a hot bath, taking care of your hygiene such as by brushing and flossing your teeth, doing a facial, applying lotion, and other activities.

Think about how babies go to sleep. Mom and Dad create a ritual around bedtime. They get a bath, a quiet story, cuddles, comfy clothing, and clean bed, and soft blankets. All of this starts well before bedtime and helps the child calm down, so that when you sit down in bed to read, they usually fall asleep fast if not with the first book, then by the third. You should do the same thing for yourself.

Do the same things nightly to help you sleep such as stretching, bathing, applying lotion, dressing for bed, and reading something positive. Bedtime is not the time to read anything upsetting, scary, or even exciting. Use that time to read uplifting or thoughtful poetry, history, or something that keeps your heart rate low.

Finally, you really need to make time for sleep. Set a daily schedule for your life and stick to it. Sleep is one of the most important factors in your schedule. You should be able to get everything you need to do done daily and still sleep at least seven to eight hours a night. It may require you to learn to say no, because it's that important to your health and your daily energy levels.

Colors and Scents That Add Pep to Your Step

One way to get more energy is to incorporate essential oils and color therapy into your life. Studies show that certain colors provide energy, while others provide calmness, and some even make you hungry. Fast food restaurants use color extensively to get you in and out fast, and movie theaters and malls often pump in the smell of popped corn or other food to get their customers to buy more food.

If it's good enough for retail, it's good enough for you. After all, they've spent the money on the studies and if it didn't work, they would have stopped doing it already.

The Right Colors for the Right Moods

Try to find ways to incorporate the right colors for the right mood you want to elicit in yourself and others into the rooms and environment that you want them to feel that way in. For example, red and violet are known as energy colors, but they may also cause problems with concentration. If you work in a high energy place, red and violet can work, but if you want to make people feel happy and productive, choose green and yellows.

Just because you want to be energetic doesn't mean everything should be red, but it may mean that the wall in the exercise room should be red. It may also mean that any room you want to relax in should be a shade of blue. This is a great color for a waiting room, for example. A soft blue that is almost white can be very soothing.

The Right Scents for the Right Moods

Scents can also make a huge difference in your energy levels. However, be cautious because some people are allergic to scents. If you're using high-quality essential oils, you may have more luck with scents for energy.

Some scents that can provide energy are:

- Orange
- Eucalyptus
- Lemon
- Cedarwood
- Grapefruit
- Peppermint
- Spearmint
- Cinnamon
- Basil
- Rosemary
- Ginger
- Thyme
- Juniper

- Neroli

The best thing to do is to buy the best essential oils you can afford and then experiment. Give each new scent at least 21 days before you make a judgment, unless it causes sinus issues or allergic reactions. Since there are so many essential oil scents that can be mood lifters and energy boosters, you have a lot to choose from. Remember, if you want to be energetic tomorrow, use something calming at night. Only use the ones above during the time that you want to feel more energetic.

How to Improve Your Energy by Staying Hydrated

In this book, hydration has been mentioned several times, but that is because it's so important. By some estimates, about 75 percent of Americans are chronically dehydrated. So many people either drink too little water, or they drink other beverages for thirst instead of water.

This is not good for us, because water affects every organ and function in your body. Whether you get headaches, suffer from sinus problems, dry skin, brittle nails, frizzy hair or something else, it may all be traced to not drinking enough water. No matter what you've heard, nothing is better for hydration than drinking regular unadulterated filtered water.

But, since even mild dehydration can cause fatigue, here are some tips to ensure that you get enough water in every single day. If at any part of the day water tastes "funny" to you even though it's fresh filtered water, try brushing your teeth because you're likely just tasting your breath instead of your water. Yes, it's true.

- Keep Water Handy – Instead of thinking that you must guzzle water, just have it handy. Keep a container of water with you always and sip it whenever you're thirsty or hungry between meals. Since most of us ignore our thirst signals, sometimes the body will signal hunger even when it's not mealtime to try to get moisture into your body.

- Drink Water Before, During and After Working Out – When you work out, you need a little extra water to replace what you lose over your basic needs. Simply drink about four ounces of water before your workout and have some to sip occasionally during your workout, and then drink another four ounces after your workout.

- Add Fruit to Your Water – If you want a change of pace, put a pitcher of water in your fridge with different types of fruit and even herbs. For example, sliced oranges and mint are good together. So are lemon and strawberry. Cucumber also makes water taste fresh and delicious and gives it a little extra something as a change of pace without adding unhealthy sugars.

- Avoid Other Beverages – Even if you enjoy coffee, coke, tea and so forth, none of these are hydrating. Make it a rule that you can only enjoy something else once you drink your mandated amount of water depending on your weight. If you must have your morning coffee, add an extra few ounces of water to your day since it's so dehydrating.

- Start and End Your Day with Fruit-Infused Water – You can even heat it up as a pick-me-up or relaxing beverage in the evening. Just choose your fruit wisely. Try mint and orange in the morning, and berries and chamomile in the evening.

- Drink Water with All Your Meals – Water needs to be the beverage of choice with meals. Some experts on digestion believe you should drink your water before and after your meal and not with it, so that your digestive juices are strong enough to digest your food. Test it out to see if it makes a difference for you.

Like most things, enough is the best, but too much is not good. Be aware of people trying to tell you to drink too much water. To calculate your needs, simply take your weight in pounds, divide by two, and then drink that many ounces of water all throughout the day. Do not guzzle water or drink water too fast, as drinking too much too fast can be very dangerous and unhealthy. Instead, make water drinking part of your daily life to enjoy all throughout the day.

Supplements That Can Help Boost Brain Power

Would it not be great if you could just pop a pill and remember everything for an exam? Realistically, there are no supplements that can boost your brain power to such astounding levels. Although, studies have shown that regular intake of certain supplements can increase the ability to memorize. There are many herbs, supplements and foods that can improve your brain; the effect of which can mean improvement of memory, learning, concentration, attention, reasoning, social skills, decision making, and focus. If you can combine these 'brain foods' with enough rest and exercise, you will have boosted your brainpower in no time.

The brain requires a variety of nutrients to produce neurotransmitters – these are substances that control mood, behavior, and mind. Studies have proved beyond doubt that nutritional supplements increase IQ and enhance learning ability. 'Smart nutrients' (cognitive-enhancing supplements) are natural substances that improve human intelligence.

Ginkgo Biloba

This substance has been used for thousands of years in Eastern cultures and is perhaps the most well-known of all memory enhancing herbs. It works by diluting the blood vessels in the brain and enhancing blood flow to the brain; thus, supplying lots of oxygen to the brain. It also gets rid of harmful free radicals that damage brain cells. However, the results are not immediate. Taking the supplement continuously for a few weeks will start yielding results.

Green Tea and Black Tea

Recent research has shown that these common constituents of the kitchen are very effective in combating the dreaded Alzheimer's disease. The most significant result seems to be that these prevent the breakdown of acetylcholine. This is a key chemical involved with memory and is lacking in Alzheimer's patients. The effect of green tea is more lasting than that of black tea, which lasts only for a day.

Sage and Rosemary

A recent study shows that students who took sage performed better at a memory recall test. Scientists believe that sage contains substances that may increase levels of a chemical that transmits messages to the brain. Rosemary also helps stimulate the memory and alleviate mental fatigue. It also strengthens mental clarity. How exactly these substances help the brain remains ambiguous.

Vitamin B Supplements

A healthy diet should provide you with all the vitamins that are needed by the body. But at times of stress and fatigue, the body gets depleted of Vitamin B. This deficiency prevents the functioning of acetylcholine. Vitamin B also helps carry oxygen to the brain and this does away with harmful free radicals. Some natural foods like liver, eggs, soybeans, lentils, and green beans are rich in Vitamin B. Vitamin B Supplements also help to boost the level of these vital vitamins in the body.

Iron deficiency

The most common deficiency in most parts of the world is linked to iron deficiency. Poor concentration, diminished intelligence, and a short attention span are all attributed to iron deficiency. Iron helps carry oxygen to the blood and its deficiency leaves the brain sadly lacking in oxygen. Iron deficiency can be detected by a simple blood test. Iron-rich food like lean meat, beans, iron-fortified cereals, and iron supplements help raise the levels of iron. But absorption of iron becomes possible only in the presence of vitamin C. Garnishing iron-rich food with lime juice is one of the most effective and natural ways to ingest Vitamin C with iron.

Water is an often overlooked but an important necessity of the brain. The brain is 70% water, and a dehydrated brain works at a slower pace. Therefore, it is necessary to keep the brain hydrated with plenty of water.

Conclusion

Recharging your body and overcoming fatigue so that you can get your life back is one of the most important ways you can improve the quality of your life. There is no reason you need to be exhausted and tired all the time. If it's not a medical condition (and even if it is), you have a lot more control over how you feel each day than you think. It might be as simple as getting enough sleep and drinking enough water. You are the one with the power to figure it out. Don't delay, so that you can get your life back and do wonderful things.

For more information, visit http://honeydbeauty.com

About the Author

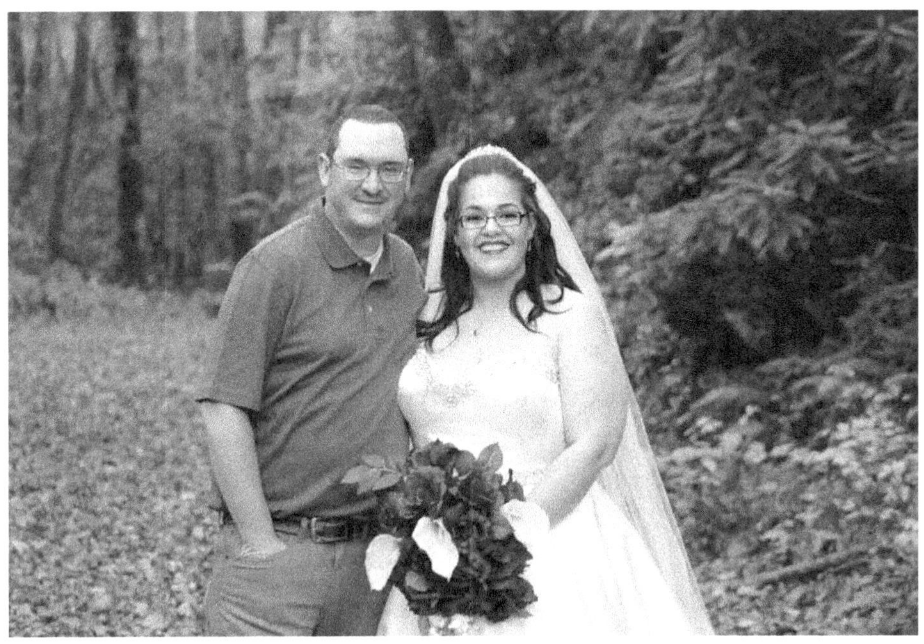

Dani lives in east Tennessee with her husband, Jonathan, and their chi-weenie, Tulip. Jonathan and Dani have been happily married for 5 years. Due to her health, Dani is unable to have children. She spends her time cuddling with her dog, who loves every moment.

Dani loves to teach and help others with their beauty and wellness needs in a holistic way. She is currently studying to become a certified health and wellness coach, as well as a life coach.

Dani has been writing for several years, which included years as a journalist for a local newspaper. She left the newspaper industry to become an entrepreneur. She now owns a beauty and wellness company, HoneyDBeauty. She helps others start their own beauty and wellness business, and works with customers to help match them with products that help them.

For more information about Dani, please visit
http://honeydbeauty.com

Follow Dani on Facebook
http://www.facebook.com/daniddyer

Follow Dani on Instagram
http://www.instagram.com/danidyer